TYPE 1 DIABETES COOKBOOK FOR BEGINNERS

BEGINNERS

Your Guide to Delicious Meals & a 30-Day Plan for Type 1 Diabetes

T. John

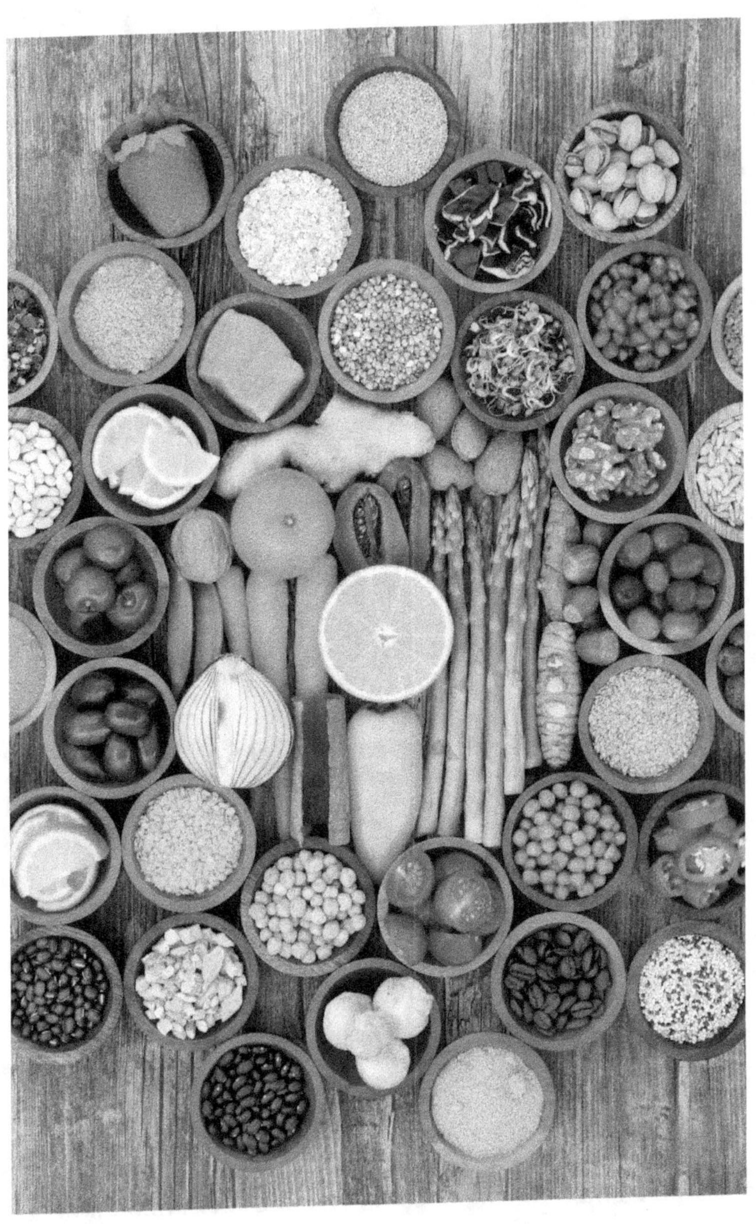

TABLE OF CONTENTS

INTRODUCTION

Type 1 diabetes, often misunderstood and shrouded in confusion, can feel like an unwelcome houseguest who just settled in. But fear not! By understanding the intricacies of this autoimmune condition and embracing a diet that empowers you, you can transform your relationship with food from one of restriction to one of informed choice and newfound freedom.

Understanding the Enemy Within:

Imagine your body as a bustling bakery. The pancreas, your resident baker, churns out insulin, the key that unlocks the doors of your cells, allowing glucose (sugar) from your meals to enter and fuel your body. In type 1 diabetes, your mischievous immune system throws a wrench in the works, mistaking insulin-producing cells for invaders and launching an attack, effectively shutting down your bakery.

The Power of Plate and Fork:

While you can't magically reopen that bakery, you can become the master chef, whipping up meals that keep your blood sugar levels dancing the hora, not the hokey-pokey. Here's how:

1. Befriend whole grains, fruits, and veggies: These rockstars are packed with fiber, slowing down the sugar parade into your bloodstream. Think brown rice instead of white, apples over sugary treats, and broccoli as your new BFF.

2. Choose lean protein sources: Chicken, fish, beans, and tofu keep you feeling satisfied without spiking your blood sugar. Grilled, baked, or steamed are your superhero sidekicks.

3. Fats? Yes, please! But the good kind, found in nuts, avocado, and olive oil. They'll keep you happy and healthy.

4. Portion control: It's not about deprivation, but mindful awareness. Use smaller plates, savor each bite, and stop when your tummy feels pleasantly content, not stuffed.

Tips for a Delicious Journey:

1. Carb counting is your compass: Learn to estimate the carbs in your food and pair them with the right insulin dose. It's like deciphering a secret recipe for perfect blood sugar harmony.

2. Be a label detective: Scan food labels like a hawk. Sugar can hide underSneaky aliases like sucrose, high-fructose corn syrup, and maltodextrin.

3. Spice up your life!: Ditch the salt shaker and add flavor with herbs, spices, and citrus. Your taste buds will thank you.

4. Plan and prep: Don't let hunger be your master. Pack healthy snacks, plan meals ahead, and involve your family. Diabetes management is a team sport!

5. Celebrate small wins: Every healthy choice is a victory lap. High five yourself for resisting that sugary temptation or trying a new veggie.

Remember: You're not alone on this culinary adventure. Lean on your healthcare team, diabetes educators, and supportive communities. With knowledge as your weapon, a positive attitude as your armor, and a willingness to experiment, you'll conquer type 1 diabetes, one delicious bite at a time!

Bonus Tip: Get creative! Explore new cuisines, rediscover old favorites with healthy twists, and turn mealtimes into a canvas for your culinary artistry. Food can be both medicine and magic; embrace its power to heal and nourish your body and soul.

Live well, eat well, and remember, with type 1 diabetes, you're not just managing a condition, you're redefining your relationship with food and becoming your own health hero!

Chapter 1: 30 Day Meal Plan

Week 1:

Day 1:

- Breakfast: Quinoa and Berry Breakfast Bowl
- Lunch: Grilled Chicken Salad with Mixed Greens
- Dinner: Baked Lemon Herb Chicken
- Snack: Hummus and Veggie Sticks
- Dessert: Berry and Yogurt Popsicles

Day 2:

- Breakfast: Avocado and Egg Breakfast Wrap
- Lunch: Quinoa and Black Bean Stuffed Peppers
- Dinner: Spaghetti Squash with Turkey Bolognese
- Snack: Guacamole with Whole Wheat Pita Chips
- Dessert: Dark Chocolate-Dipped Strawberries

Day 3:

- Breakfast: Greek Yogurt Parfait with Nuts and Berries
- Lunch: Turkey and Veggie Wrap with Hummus

- Dinner: Teriyaki Glazed Salmon with Quinoa

- Snack: Greek Yogurt and Berry Parfait

- Dessert: Banana and Walnut Muffins

Day 4:

- Breakfast: Chia Seed Pudding with Almond Milk

- Lunch: Lentil and Vegetable Soup

- Dinner: Cauliflower Crust Pizza with Veggies

- Snack: Almond and Date Energy Balls

- Dessert: Greek Yogurt and Honey Frozen Cups

Day 5:

- Breakfast: Oatmeal with Fresh Fruit and Cinnamon

- Lunch: Grilled Shrimp and Quinoa Bowl

- Dinner: Black Bean and Vegetable Enchiladas

- Snack: Edamame with Sea Salt

- Dessert: Baked Apple with Cinnamon

Day 6:

- Breakfast: Veggie Omelette with Whole Grain Toast

- Lunch: Chickpea and Vegetable Stir-Fry

- Dinner: Garlic and Herb Roasted Vegetables with Tofu
- Snack: Veggie and Cheese Skewers
- Dessert: Avocado Chocolate Mousse

Day 7:

- Breakfast: Spinach and Feta Breakfast Muffins
- Lunch: Caprese Salad with Balsamic Glaze
- Dinner: Stuffed Bell Peppers with Ground Turkey
- Snack: Cottage Cheese and Pineapple Salsa
- Dessert: Almond Flour Blueberry Cookies

Week 2:

Day 8:

- Breakfast: Sweet Potato Hash with Poached Eggs
- Lunch: Zucchini Noodles with Pesto and Cherry Tomatoes
- Dinner: Shrimp and Vegetable Stir-Fry with Brown Rice
- Snack: Apple Slices with Nut Butter
- Dessert: Mango and Coconut Chia Pudding

Day 9:

- Breakfast: Cottage Cheese Pancakes
- Lunch: Tofu and Broccoli Quinoa Bowl
- Dinner: Lemon Garlic Tilapia with Asparagus
- Snack: Roasted Chickpeas with Cumin
- Dessert: Pumpkin Pie Smoothie

Day 10:

- Breakfast: Nut Butter Banana Toast
- Lunch: Chicken and Vegetable Skewers with Brown Rice
- Dinner: Quinoa and Vegetable Casserole
- Snack: Caprese Skewers with Balsamic Glaze
- Dessert: Mixed Berry Sorbet

Day 11:

- Breakfast: Breakfast Burrito with Black Beans and Salsa
- Lunch: Greek Salad with Feta and Olives
- Dinner: Chicken and Broccoli Alfredo with Whole Wheat Pasta
- Snack: Trail Mix with Nuts and Dried Fruit

- Dessert: Quinoa and Berry Parfait

Day 12:

- Breakfast: Smoked Salmon and Cream Cheese Bagel
- Lunch: Sweet Potato and Kale Salad
- Dinner: Mediterranean Stuffed Chicken Breast
- Snack: Whole Grain Crackers with Smoked Salmon
- Dessert: Cinnamon Baked Pears

Day 13:

- Breakfast: Blueberry Almond Smoothie Bowl
- Lunch: Salmon and Asparagus Foil Pack
- Dinner: Sweet and Sour Tofu with Cauliflower Rice
- Snack: Kale Chips with Parmesan
- Dessert: Coconut Flour Chocolate Cake

Day 14:

- Breakfast: Apple Cinnamon Quinoa Porridge
- Lunch: Egg Salad Lettuce Wraps
- Dinner: Turkey and Sweet Potato Chili
- Snack: Greek Salad Lettuce Wraps
- Dessert: Peanut Butter and Banana Ice Cream

Week 3:

Day 15:

- Breakfast: Tomato and Basil Breakfast Frittata
- Lunch: Spinach and Mushroom Quesadilla
- Dinner: BBQ Grilled Veggie Skewers
- Snack: Mini Turkey and Quinoa Meatballs
- Dessert: Lemon Poppy Seed Energy Bites

Day 16:

- Breakfast: Quinoa and Berry Breakfast Bowl
- Lunch: Grilled Chicken Salad with Mixed Greens
- Dinner: Baked Lemon Herb Chicken
- Snack: Hummus and Veggie Sticks
- Dessert: Berry and Yogurt Popsicles

Day 17:

- Breakfast: Avocado and Egg Breakfast Wrap
- Lunch: Quinoa and Black Bean Stuffed Peppers
- Dinner: Spaghetti Squash with Turkey Bolognese
- Snack: Guacamole with Whole Wheat Pita Chips
- Dessert: Dark Chocolate-Dipped Strawberries

Day 18:

- Breakfast: Greek Yogurt Parfait with Nuts and Berries
- Lunch: Turkey and Veggie Wrap with Hummus
- Dinner: Teriyaki Glazed Salmon with Quinoa
- Snack: Greek Yogurt and Berry Parfait
- Dessert: Banana and Walnut Muffins

Day 19:

- Breakfast: Chia Seed Pudding with Almond Milk
- Lunch: Lentil and Vegetable Soup
- Dinner: Cauliflower Crust Pizza with Veggies
- Snack: Almond and Date Energy Balls
- Dessert: Greek Yogurt and Honey Frozen Cups

Day 20:

- Breakfast: Oatmeal with Fresh Fruit and Cinnamon
- Lunch: Grilled Shrimp and Quinoa Bowl
- Dinner: Black Bean and Vegetable Enchiladas
- Snack: Edamame with Sea Salt
- Dessert: Baked Apple with Cinnamon

Day 21:

- Breakfast: Veggie Omelette with Whole Grain Toast
- Lunch: Chickpea and Vegetable Stir-Fry
- Dinner: Garlic and Herb Roasted Vegetables with Tofu
- Snack: Veggie and Cheese Skewers
- Dessert: Avocado Chocolate Mousse

Week 4:

Day 22:

- Breakfast: Spinach and Feta Breakfast Muffins
- Lunch: Caprese Salad with Balsamic Glaze
- Dinner: Stuffed Bell Peppers with Ground Turkey
- Snack: Cottage Cheese and Pineapple Salsa
- Dessert: Almond Flour Blueberry Cookies

Day 23:

- Breakfast: Sweet Potato Hash with Poached Eggs
- Lunch: Zucchini Noodles with Pesto and Cherry Tomatoes
- Dinner: Shrimp and Vegetable Stir-Fry with Brown Rice

- Snack: Apple Slices with Nut Butter

- Dessert: Mango and Coconut Chia Pudding

Day 24:

- Breakfast: Cottage Cheese Pancakes

- Lunch: Tofu and Broccoli Quinoa Bowl

- Dinner: Lemon Garlic Tilapia with Asparagus

- Snack: Roasted Chickpeas with Cumin

- Dessert: Pumpkin Pie Smoothie

Day 25:

- Breakfast: Nut Butter Banana Toast

- Lunch: Chicken and Vegetable Skewers with Brown Rice

- Dinner: Quinoa and Vegetable Casserole

- Snack: Caprese Skewers with Balsamic Glaze

- Dessert: Mixed Berry Sorbet

Day 26:

- Breakfast: Breakfast Burrito with Black Beans and Salsa

- Lunch: Greek Salad with Feta and Olives

- Dinner: Chicken and Broccoli Alfredo with Whole Wheat Pasta
- Snack: Trail Mix with Nuts and Dried Fruit
- Dessert: Quinoa and Berry Parfait

Day 27:

- Breakfast: Smoked Salmon and Cream Cheese Bagel
- Lunch: Sweet Potato and Kale Salad
- Dinner: Mediterranean Stuffed Chicken Breast
- Snack: Whole Grain Crackers with Smoked Salmon
- Dessert: Cinnamon Baked Pears

Day 28:

- Breakfast: Blueberry Almond Smoothie Bowl
- Lunch: Salmon and Asparagus Foil Pack
- Dinner: Sweet and Sour Tofu with Cauliflower Rice
- Snack: Kale Chips with Parmesan
- Dessert: Coconut Flour Chocolate Cake

Day 29:

- Breakfast: Apple Cinnamon Quinoa Porridge
- Lunch: Egg Salad Lettuce Wraps

- Dinner: Turkey and Sweet Potato Chili

- Snack: Greek Salad Lettuce Wraps

- Dessert: Peanut Butter and Banana Ice Cream

Day 30:

- Breakfast: Tomato and Basil Breakfast Frittata

- Lunch: Spinach and Mushroom Quesadilla

- Dinner: BBQ Grilled Veggie Skewers

- Snack: Mini Turkey and Quinoa Meatballs

- Dessert: Lemon Poppy Seed Energy Bites

Chapter 2: Breakfast Recipes

In this chapter, we've curated a collection of wholesome breakfast recipes that not only cater to your taste buds but also prioritize your health. From hearty bowls to satisfying wraps, these recipes are designed to provide the right balance of nutrients to kickstart your morning.

Quinoa and Berry Breakfast Bowl

Ingredients:

- 1/2 cup quinoa, cooked
- 1/2 cup mixed berries (strawberries, blueberries, raspberries)
- 1 tablespoon honey
- 1 tablespoon chopped almonds
- 1/2 cup Greek yogurt

Instructions:

1. In a bowl, layer cooked quinoa.
2. Top with mixed berries and drizzle honey.
3. Sprinkle chopped almonds over the berries.

4. Add a dollop of Greek yogurt.

5. Gently mix and enjoy!

Nutrition Information:

- Calories: 300

- Protein: 15g

- Carbohydrates: 45g

- Fat: 8g

- Fiber: 6g

- Sugar: 15g

- Portion Size: 1 bowl

Avocado and Egg Breakfast Wrap

Ingredients:

- 1 whole wheat tortilla

- 1/2 avocado, sliced

- 2 eggs, scrambled

- Salt and pepper to taste

- Fresh cilantro (optional)

Instructions:

1. Warm the tortilla in a pan.

2. Layer sliced avocado on the tortilla.

3. Scramble eggs with salt and pepper; place on the avocado.

4. Garnish with fresh cilantro if desired.

5. Roll into a wrap and enjoy!

Nutrition Information:

- Calories: 350
- Protein: 18g
- Carbohydrates: 25g
- Fat: 20g
- Fiber: 8g
- Sugar: 2g
- Portion Size: 1 wrap

Greek Yogurt Parfait with Nuts and Berries

Ingredients:

- 1 cup Greek yogurt
- 1/2 cup mixed berries
- 2 tablespoons granola

- 1 tablespoon chopped nuts

- Honey for drizzling

Instructions:

1. In a glass, layer Greek yogurt.

2. Add mixed berries and sprinkle granola.

3. Top with chopped nuts.

4. Drizzle honey over the parfait.

5. Repeat the layers and savor!

Nutrition Information:

- Calories: 280

- Protein: 20g

- Carbohydrates: 30g

- Fat: 10g

- Fiber: 4g

- Sugar: 15g

- Portion Size: 1 parfait

Chia Seed Pudding with Almond Milk

Ingredients:

- 2 tablespoons chia seeds

- 1 cup unsweetened almond milk
- 1/2 teaspoon vanilla extract
- 1 tablespoon maple syrup
- Fresh fruit for topping

Instructions:

1. In a jar, mix chia seeds, almond milk, vanilla extract, and maple syrup.
2. Stir well and refrigerate overnight.
3. Before serving, top with fresh fruit.
4. Stir once more and enjoy the pudding!

Nutrition Information:

- Calories: 180
- Protein: 5g
- Carbohydrates: 20g
- Fat: 10g
- Fiber: 8g
- Sugar: 7g
- Portion Size: 1 serving

Oatmeal with Fresh Fruit and Cinnamon

Ingredients:

- 1/2 cup rolled oats
- 1 cup water or milk
- 1/2 banana, sliced
- Handful of berries
- 1/2 teaspoon cinnamon

Instructions:

1. Cook oats with water or milk according to package instructions.
2. Top with banana slices and berries.
3. Sprinkle with cinnamon.
4. Mix well and savor the warm goodness!

Nutrition Information:

- Calories: 220
- Protein: 7g
- Carbohydrates: 40g
- Fat: 4g
- Fiber: 6g

- Sugar: 8g
- Portion Size: 1 bowl

Veggie Omelette with Whole Grain Toast

Ingredients:

- 2 eggs, beaten
- Bell peppers, onions, and tomatoes (diced)
- Handful of spinach
- Salt and pepper to taste
- 1 slice whole grain bread, toasted

Instructions:

1. In a pan, sauté veggies until tender.
2. Pour beaten eggs over veggies; cook until set.
3. Fold the omelette and season with salt and pepper.
4. Serve with a slice of toasted whole grain bread.

Nutrition Information:

- Calories: 250
- Protein: 15g

- Carbohydrates: 20g

- Fat: 12g

- Fiber: 5g

- Sugar: 3g

- Portion Size: 1 serving

Spinach and Feta Breakfast Muffins

Ingredients:

- 2 cups fresh spinach, chopped

- 1/2 cup feta cheese, crumbled

- 4 eggs

- 1/4 cup milk

- Salt and pepper to taste

Instructions:

1. Preheat oven to 350°F (175°C).

2. In a bowl, mix spinach and feta.

3. In another bowl, whisk eggs, milk, salt, and pepper.

4. Combine the egg mixture with spinach and feta.

5. Pour into muffin cups and bake for 20-25 minutes.

Nutrition Information:

- Calories: 180
- Protein: 14g
- Carbohydrates: 4g
- Fat: 12g
- Fiber: 2g
- Sugar: 2g
- Portion Size: 2 muffins

Sweet Potato Hash with Poached Eggs

Ingredients:

- 1 sweet potato, diced
- 2 eggs
- 1/2 onion, finely chopped
- 1 bell pepper, diced
- 1 tablespoon olive oil
- Salt and pepper to taste

Instructions:

1. In a pan, sauté sweet potatoes, onions, and bell peppers in olive oil.
2. Season with salt and pepper.
3. Poach eggs and place on top of the hash.
4. Serve warm and enjoy this savory breakfast!

Nutrition Information:

- Calories: 280
- Protein: 12g
- Carbohydrates: 30g
- Fat: 14g
- Fiber: 6g
- Sugar: 8g
- Portion Size: 1 serving

Cottage Cheese Pancakes

Ingredients:

- 1/2 cup cottage cheese
- 2 eggs
- 1/4 cup almond flour
- 1/2 teaspoon vanilla extract

- Berries for topping

Instructions:

1. Blend cottage cheese, eggs, almond flour, and vanilla until smooth.
2. Heat a skillet and pour small pancake-sized portions.
3. Cook until bubbles form, then flip.
4. Top with berries and enjoy these protein-packed pancakes!

Nutrition Information:

- Calories: 220
- Protein: 15g
- Carbohydrates: 10g
- Fat: 12g
- Fiber: 2g
- Sugar: 4g
- Portion Size: 2 pancakes

Nut Butter Banana Toast

Ingredients:

- 1 slice whole grain bread, toasted

- 2 tablespoons nut butter (almond, peanut, or your choice)
- 1 banana, sliced
- Drizzle of honey

Instructions:

1. Spread nut butter on the toasted bread.
2. Arrange banana slices on top.
3. Drizzle with honey.
4. A simple, yet satisfying breakfast is ready!

Nutrition Information:

- Calories: 280
- Protein: 8g
- Carbohydrates: 35g
- Fat: 14g
- Fiber: 6g
- Sugar: 15g
- Portion Size: 1 serving

Breakfast Burrito with Black Beans and Salsa

Ingredients:

- 1 whole wheat tortilla
- 1/2 cup black beans, cooked
- 2 eggs, scrambled
- Salsa and avocado for topping
- Fresh cilantro (optional)

Instructions:

1. Warm the tortilla in a pan.
2. Layer black beans and scrambled eggs.
3. Top with salsa and sliced avocado.
4. Garnish with fresh cilantro if desired.
5. Roll into a burrito and savor the flavors!

Nutrition Information:

- Calories: 320
- Protein: 18g
- Carbohydrates: 35g
- Fat: 14g
- Fiber: 10g

- Sugar: 3g
- Portion Size: 1 burrito

Smoked Salmon and Cream Cheese Bagel

Ingredients:

- 1 whole grain or multigrain bagel, toasted
- 2 ounces smoked salmon
- 2 tablespoons cream cheese
- Sliced cucumber and red onion

Instructions:

1. Spread cream cheese on the toasted bagel halves.
2. Layer with smoked salmon, cucumber, and red onion slices.
3. Close the bagel and relish this classic combination!

Nutrition Information:

- Calories: 350
- Protein: 20g
- Carbohydrates: 40g

- Fat: 14g

- Fiber: 5g

- Sugar: 5g

- Portion Size: 1 bagel sandwich

Blueberry Almond Smoothie Bowl

Ingredients:

- 1 cup frozen blueberries

- 1/2 banana, frozen

- 1/2 cup almond milk

- 1 tablespoon almond butter

- Toppings: Granola, sliced almonds, and fresh blueberries

Instructions:

1. Blend frozen blueberries, frozen banana, almond milk, and almond butter until smooth.

2. Pour into a bowl and top with granola, sliced almonds, and fresh blueberries.

3. Dive into this refreshing and nutrient-packed bowl!

Nutrition Information:

- Calories: 290
- Protein: 8g
- Carbohydrates: 40g
- Fat: 12g
- Fiber: 10g
- Sugar: 20g
- Portion Size: 1 bowl

Apple Cinnamon Quinoa Porridge

Ingredients:

- 1/2 cup quinoa, rinsed
- 1 cup unsweetened almond milk
- 1 apple, diced
- 1/2 teaspoon cinnamon
- 1 tablespoon maple syrup

Instructions:

1. Cook quinoa in almond milk according to package instructions.
2. Add diced apple, cinnamon, and maple syrup.
3. Simmer until the apple is tender.

4. Enjoy a warm and comforting quinoa porridge!

Nutrition Information:

- Calories: 260

- Protein: 7g

- Carbohydrates: 45g

- Fat: 5g

- Fiber: 6g

- Sugar: 18g

- Portion Size: 1 serving

Tomato and Basil Breakfast Frittata

Ingredients:

- 4 eggs, beaten

- 1 cup cherry tomatoes, halved

- Fresh basil leaves, chopped

- 1/4 cup feta cheese, crumbled

- Salt and pepper to taste

Instructions:

1. Preheat oven to 350°F (175°C).

2. Mix beaten eggs with cherry tomatoes, basil, and feta.

3. Season with salt and pepper.

4. Pour into a greased baking dish and bake for 20-25 minutes.

5. Slice into wedges and savor this flavorful frittata!

Nutrition Information:

- Calories: 220
- Protein: 14g
- Carbohydrates: 5g
- Fat: 16g
- Fiber: 2g
- Sugar: 3g
- Portion Size: 1 serving

Chapter 3: Lunch Recipes

These recipes are carefully crafted with wholesome ingredients, ensuring a balance of flavors and health benefits. Each recipe is numbered and comes with detailed instructions, making it easy for beginners to create delicious and diabetes-friendly lunches. Let's dive into the culinary adventure!

Grilled Chicken Salad with Mixed Greens

Ingredients:

- 2 boneless, skinless chicken breasts
- 4 cups mixed salad greens
- 1 cup cherry tomatoes, halved
- 1 cucumber, sliced
- 1/4 cup red onion, thinly sliced
- 2 tablespoons olive oil
- 1 tablespoon balsamic vinegar
- Salt and pepper to taste

Instructions:

1. Preheat the grill to medium-high heat.
2. Season chicken breasts with salt and pepper.
3. Grill chicken for 6-8 minutes per side or until fully cooked.
4. In a large bowl, combine salad greens, cherry tomatoes, cucumber, and red onion.
5. Slice grilled chicken and place on top of the salad.
6. In a small bowl, whisk together olive oil and balsamic vinegar.
7. Drizzle dressing over the salad and toss gently.
8. Serve immediately.

Nutrition Information:

- Calories: 350
- Protein: 30g
- Carbohydrates: 10g
- Fat: 20g
- Fiber: 4g
- Sugar: 4g
- Portion Size: 1 serving

Quinoa and Black Bean Stuffed Peppers

Ingredients:

- 4 bell peppers, halved and seeds removed
- 1 cup cooked quinoa
- 1 can (15 oz) black beans, drained and rinsed
- 1 cup corn kernels
- 1 cup diced tomatoes
- 1 teaspoon cumin
- 1 teaspoon chili powder
- Salt and pepper to taste
- 1 cup shredded cheddar cheese (optional)

Instructions:

1. Preheat the oven to 375°F (190°C).
2. In a large bowl, mix together quinoa, black beans, corn, diced tomatoes, cumin, chili powder, salt, and pepper.
3. Spoon the mixture into halved bell peppers.
4. Place stuffed peppers in a baking dish.
5. If desired, sprinkle shredded cheddar cheese on top.
6. Bake for 25-30 minutes or until peppers are tender.

7. Remove from the oven and let it cool for a few minutes before serving.

Nutrition Information:

- Calories: 280
- Protein: 12g
- Carbohydrates: 45g
- Fat: 5g
- Fiber: 10g
- Sugar: 8g
- Portion Size: 2 halves

Turkey and Veggie Wrap with Hummus

Ingredients:

- 4 whole-grain wraps
- 1 pound lean ground turkey
- 1 cup mixed vegetables (bell peppers, zucchini, carrots), chopped
- 1 teaspoon garlic powder
- 1 teaspoon onion powder

- Salt and pepper to taste
- 1/2 cup hummus

Instructions:

1. In a skillet over medium heat, cook ground turkey until browned.
2. Add mixed vegetables and cook until tender.
3. Season with garlic powder, onion powder, salt, and pepper.
4. Warm the whole-grain wraps in a dry pan.
5. Spread hummus on each wrap.
6. Spoon turkey and vegetable mixture onto each wrap.
7. Fold in the sides and roll up the wraps.
8. Slice in half and serve.

Nutrition Information:

- Calories: 320
- Protein: 25g
- Carbohydrates: 30g
- Fat: 12g
- Fiber: 6g
- Sugar: 3g

- Portion Size: 1 wrap

Lentil and Vegetable Soup

Ingredients:

- 1 cup dried green lentils, rinsed
- 1 onion, diced
- 2 carrots, sliced
- 2 celery stalks, chopped
- 3 cloves garlic, minced
- 1 can (14 oz) diced tomatoes
- 6 cups vegetable broth
- 1 teaspoon dried thyme
- 1 teaspoon cumin
- Salt and pepper to taste

Instructions:

1. In a large pot, combine lentils, onion, carrots, celery, garlic, diced tomatoes, vegetable broth, thyme, cumin, salt, and pepper.
2. Bring to a boil, then reduce heat and simmer for 25-30 minutes or until lentils are tender.
3. Adjust seasoning if needed before serving.

Nutrition Information:

- Calories: 220
- Protein: 14g
- Carbohydrates: 40g
- Fat: 1g
- Fiber: 15g
- Sugar: 6g
- Portion Size: 1.5 cups

Grilled Shrimp and Quinoa Bowl

Ingredients:

- 1 cup quinoa, cooked
- 1 pound shrimp, peeled and deveined
- 1 tablespoon olive oil
- 1 teaspoon paprika
- 1 teaspoon garlic powder
- Salt and pepper to taste
- 1 cup broccoli florets, steamed
- 1/2 cup cherry tomatoes, halved
- 1/4 cup feta cheese (optional)

Instructions:

1. In a bowl, toss shrimp with olive oil, paprika, garlic powder, salt, and pepper.
2. Grill shrimp for 2-3 minutes per side or until cooked through.
3. Assemble the bowl with quinoa, grilled shrimp, steamed broccoli, and cherry tomatoes.
4. Sprinkle with feta cheese if desired.

Nutrition Information:

- Calories: 330
- Protein: 30g
- Carbohydrates: 30g
- Fat: 10g
- Fiber: 5g
- Sugar: 3g
- Portion Size: 1 bowl

Chickpea and Vegetable Stir-Fry

Ingredients:

- 1 can (15 oz) chickpeas, drained and rinsed

- 2 cups mixed vegetables (bell peppers, broccoli, snap peas)
- 2 tablespoons soy sauce
- 1 tablespoon sesame oil
- 1 teaspoon ginger, grated
- 2 cloves garlic, minced
- 1 tablespoon rice vinegar
- 1 tablespoon sesame seeds (optional)

Instructions:

1. In a wok or large skillet, heat sesame oil over medium-high heat.
2. Add mixed vegetables and stir-fry for 3-4 minutes until tender-crisp.
3. Add chickpeas and continue to stir-fry for an additional 2-3 minutes.
4. In a small bowl, whisk together soy sauce, ginger, garlic, and rice vinegar.
5. Pour the sauce over the stir-fry and toss to coat.
6. Sprinkle with sesame seeds if desired before serving.

Nutrition Information:

- Calories: 250
- Protein: 10g
- Carbohydrates: 35g
- Fat: 8g
- Fiber: 8g
- Sugar: 8g
- Portion Size: 1.5 cups

Caprese Salad with Balsamic Glaze

Ingredients:

- 4 large tomatoes, sliced
- 1 pound fresh mozzarella, sliced
- Fresh basil leaves
- 2 tablespoons balsamic glaze
- Salt and pepper to taste

Instructions:

1. Arrange tomato and mozzarella slices on a serving platter.
2. Tuck fresh basil leaves between the slices.
3. Drizzle balsamic glaze over the salad.

4. Sprinkle with salt and pepper to taste.

Nutrition Information:

- Calories: 280
- Protein: 18g
- Carbohydrates: 10g
- Fat: 20g
- Fiber: 2g
- Sugar: 6g
- Portion Size: 1 serving

Zucchini Noodles with Pesto and Cherry Tomatoes

Ingredients:

- 4 medium zucchinis, spiralized
- 1 cup cherry tomatoes, halved
- 1/2 cup basil pesto (store-bought or homemade)
- 1/4 cup pine nuts, toasted
- Parmesan cheese for garnish (optional)

Instructions:

1. In a large pan, sauté zucchini noodles over medium heat until just tender.
2. Toss zucchini noodles with cherry tomatoes and basil pesto.
3. Sprinkle with toasted pine nuts.
4. Garnish with Parmesan cheese if desired.

Nutrition Information:

- Calories: 320
- Protein: 8g
- Carbohydrates: 15g
- Fat: 25g
- Fiber: 5g
- Sugar: 6g
- Portion Size: 1.5 cups

Tofu and Broccoli Quinoa Bowl

Ingredients:

- 1 cup quinoa, cooked
- 1 block firm tofu, cubed
- 2 cups broccoli florets

- 2 tablespoons soy sauce
- 1 tablespoon sesame oil
- 1 teaspoon garlic powder
- 1 teaspoon ginger, grated
- 1 tablespoon rice vinegar
- Green onions for garnish

Instructions:

1. In a large skillet, heat sesame oil over medium heat.
2. Add tofu cubes and cook until golden brown on all sides.
3. Steam broccoli until tender-crisp.
4. In a bowl, combine cooked quinoa, tofu, and broccoli.
5. In a small bowl, whisk together soy sauce, garlic powder, ginger, and rice vinegar.
6. Pour the sauce over the quinoa mixture and toss to coat.
7. Garnish with green onions before serving.

Nutrition Information:

- Calories: 380

- Protein: 20g

- Carbohydrates: 40g

- Fat: 15g

- Fiber: 8g

- Sugar: 2g

- Portion Size: 1 bowl

Chicken and Vegetable Skewers with Brown Rice

Ingredients:

- 1 pound chicken breast, cut into cubes

- 2 bell peppers, cut into chunks

- 1 red onion, cut into chunks

- 2 tablespoons olive oil

- 1 teaspoon dried oregano

- 1 teaspoon paprika

- Salt and pepper to taste

- 2 cups brown rice, cooked

Instructions:

1. Preheat grill or grill pan to medium-high heat.

2. In a bowl, toss chicken, bell peppers, and red onion with olive oil, oregano, paprika, salt, and pepper.

3. Thread the chicken and vegetables onto skewers.

4. Grill skewers for 8-10 minutes, turning occasionally, until chicken is cooked through.

5. Serve skewers over a bed of cooked brown rice.

Nutrition Information:

- Calories: 420
- Protein: 30g
- Carbohydrates: 40g
- Fat: 15g
- Fiber: 5g
- Sugar: 3g
- Portion Size: 1 serving

Greek Salad with Feta and Olives

Ingredients:

- 4 cups mixed salad greens
- 1 cup cherry tomatoes, halved
- 1 cucumber, sliced
- 1/2 cup Kalamata olives, pitted

- 1/2 cup feta cheese, crumbled

- 2 tablespoons olive oil

- 1 tablespoon red wine vinegar

- 1 teaspoon dried oregano

- Salt and pepper to taste

Instructions:

1. In a large bowl, combine salad greens, cherry tomatoes, cucumber, olives, and feta cheese.

2. In a small bowl, whisk together olive oil, red wine vinegar, oregano, salt, and pepper.

3. Drizzle the dressing over the salad and toss gently.

4. Serve immediately.

Nutrition Information:

- Calories: 280

- Protein: 8g

- Carbohydrates: 15g

- Fat: 20g

- Fiber: 5g

- Sugar: 4g

- Portion Size: 1 serving

Sweet Potato and Kale Salad

Ingredients:

- 2 sweet potatoes, peeled and cubed
- 4 cups kale, chopped
- 1/2 cup pecans, toasted
- 1/4 cup dried cranberries
- 2 tablespoons olive oil
- 1 tablespoon maple syrup
- 1 tablespoon balsamic vinegar
- Salt and pepper to taste

Instructions:

1. Preheat the oven to 400°F (200°C).
2. Toss sweet potato cubes with olive oil, maple syrup, salt, and pepper.
3. Roast sweet potatoes for 20-25 minutes or until tender.
4. In a large bowl, massage kale with balsamic vinegar until slightly wilted.
5. Add roasted sweet potatoes, toasted pecans, and dried cranberries to the kale.
6. Toss gently and serve.

Nutrition Information:

- Calories: 320
- Protein: 6g
- Carbohydrates: 45g
- Fat: 15g
- Fiber: 8g
- Sugar: 15g
- Portion Size: 1.5 cups

Salmon and Asparagus Foil Pack

Ingredients:

- 4 salmon fillets
- 1 bunch asparagus, trimmed
- 2 tablespoons olive oil
- 2 cloves garlic, minced
- 1 teaspoon lemon zest
- 1 tablespoon lemon juice
- 1 teaspoon dried dill
- Salt and pepper to taste

Instructions:

1. Preheat the oven to 400°F (200°C).

2. Place each salmon fillet on a piece of foil.

3. Arrange asparagus around the salmon.

4. In a small bowl, mix together olive oil, garlic, lemon zest, lemon juice, dried dill, salt, and pepper.

5. Drizzle the mixture over the salmon and asparagus.

6. Seal the foil packs and bake for 15-20 minutes or until salmon is cooked through.

Nutrition Information:

- Calories: 380
- Protein: 30g
- Carbohydrates: 10g
- Fat: 25g
- Fiber: 5g
- Sugar: 3g
- Portion Size: 1 foil pack

Egg Salad Lettuce Wraps

Ingredients:

- 6 hard-boiled eggs, chopped
- 1/4 cup Greek yogurt
- 1 tablespoon Dijon mustard

- 2 green onions, chopped
- Salt and pepper to taste
- Lettuce leaves for wrapping

Instructions:

1. In a bowl, combine chopped eggs, Greek yogurt, Dijon mustard, green onions, salt, and pepper.
2. Mix until well combined.
3. Spoon the egg salad onto lettuce leaves.
4. Wrap and secure with toothpicks if needed.
5. Serve chilled.

Nutrition Information:

- Calories: 250
- Protein: 20g
- Carbohydrates: 5g
- Fat: 16g
- Fiber: 2g
- Sugar: 3g
- Portion Size: 2 wraps

Spinach and Mushroom Quesadilla

Ingredients:

- 4 whole wheat tortillas
- 2 cups spinach, chopped
- 1 cup mushrooms, sliced
- 1 cup shredded mozzarella cheese
- 1 tablespoon olive oil
- 1 teaspoon garlic powder
- Salt and pepper to taste

Instructions:

1. In a skillet, sauté spinach and mushrooms in olive oil until wilted.
2. Season with garlic powder, salt, and pepper.
3. Place a tortilla in the skillet, add a layer of cheese, followed by the spinach-mushroom mixture.
4. Top with another layer of cheese and place another tortilla on top.
5. Cook until the tortilla is golden brown, then flip and cook the other side.
6. Repeat for the remaining quesadillas.
7. Slice and serve.

Nutrition Information:

- Calories: 320
- Protein: 15g
- Carbohydrates: 40g
- Fat: 12g
- Fiber: 6g
- Sugar: 2g
- Portion Size: 1 quesadilla

Chapter 4: Dinner Recipes

In this Chapter, we bring you a collection of dinner recipes that not only cater to your nutritional needs but also tantalize your taste buds. From succulent proteins to wholesome grains and vibrant vegetables, each recipe is thoughtfully crafted to strike the perfect balance..

Baked Lemon Herb Chicken

Ingredients:

- 4 boneless, skinless chicken breasts
- 2 tablespoons olive oil
- 1 lemon (juiced)
- 2 cloves garlic (minced)
- 1 teaspoon dried thyme
- 1 teaspoon dried rosemary
- Salt and pepper to taste

Instructions:

1. Preheat the oven to 375°F (190°C).

2. In a small bowl, mix olive oil, lemon juice, minced garlic, dried thyme, dried rosemary, salt, and pepper.

3. Place chicken breasts in a baking dish and pour the lemon herb mixture over them.

4. Bake for 25-30 minutes or until chicken is cooked through.

5. Serve with a side of steamed vegetables.

Nutrition Information:

- Calories: 250

- Protein: 30g

- Carbohydrates: 2g

- Fat: 14g

- Fiber: 0.5g

- Sugar: 0.5g

- Portion Size: 1 chicken breast

Spaghetti Squash with Turkey Bolognese

Ingredients:

- 1 medium spaghetti squash

- 1 pound ground turkey
- 1 onion (chopped)
- 2 cloves garlic (minced)
- 1 can (14 oz) crushed tomatoes
- 1 teaspoon dried oregano
- 1 teaspoon dried basil
- Salt and pepper to taste

Instructions:

1. Preheat the oven to 375°F (190°C).
2. Cut the spaghetti squash in half, scoop out the seeds, and place it cut side down on a baking sheet. Bake for 40-45 minutes.
3. In a skillet, cook ground turkey, chopped onion, and minced garlic until turkey is browned.
4. Add crushed tomatoes, dried oregano, dried basil, salt, and pepper to the skillet. Simmer for 15-20 minutes.
5. Scrape the cooked spaghetti squash with a fork to create "noodles." Top with turkey Bolognese sauce.

Nutrition Information:

- Calories: 320
- Protein: 25g
- Carbohydrates: 20g
- Fat: 15g
- Fiber: 5g
- Sugar: 8g
- Portion Size: 1 cup

Teriyaki Glazed Salmon with Quinoa

Ingredients:

- 4 salmon fillets
- 1/4 cup low-sodium soy sauce
- 2 tablespoons honey
- 1 tablespoon rice vinegar
- 1 teaspoon grated ginger
- 2 cloves garlic (minced)
- 1 cup cooked quinoa
- Sesame seeds and green onions for garnish

Instructions:

1. Preheat the oven to 400°F (200°C).

2. In a bowl, mix soy sauce, honey, rice vinegar, grated ginger, and minced garlic to create the teriyaki glaze.

3. Place salmon fillets on a baking sheet and brush with teriyaki glaze. Bake for 15-20 minutes.

4. Serve salmon over a bed of cooked quinoa, garnished with sesame seeds and chopped green onions.

Nutrition Information:

- Calories: 350
- Protein: 25g
- Carbohydrates: 30g
- Fat: 15g
- Fiber: 3g
- Sugar: 10g
- Portion Size: 1 salmon fillet with quinoa

Cauliflower Crust Pizza with Veggies

Ingredients:

- 1 cauliflower head (riced)
- 1 cup mozzarella cheese (shredded)

- 1 egg
- 1 teaspoon dried oregano
- 1/2 teaspoon garlic powder
- 1/4 cup tomato sauce
- Assorted vegetables (bell peppers, cherry tomatoes, mushrooms)
- Fresh basil for garnish

Instructions:

1. Preheat the oven to 425°F (220°C).
2. Mix riced cauliflower, shredded mozzarella, egg, dried oregano, and garlic powder to form the pizza crust.
3. Press the crust onto a baking sheet and bake for 15-20 minutes until golden.
4. Spread tomato sauce on the crust and top with sliced vegetables. Bake for an additional 10 minutes.
5. Garnish with fresh basil before serving.

Nutrition Information:

- Calories: 220
- Protein: 15g

- Carbohydrates: 20g

- Fat: 10g

- Fiber: 6g

- Sugar: 5g

- Portion Size: 2 slices

Black Bean and Vegetable Enchiladas

Ingredients:

- 1 can (15 oz) black beans (rinsed and drained)

- 1 cup corn kernels

- 1 bell pepper (diced)

- 1 zucchini (diced)

- 1 cup enchilada sauce

- 8 whole-grain tortillas

- 1 cup shredded cheese (cheddar or Mexican blend)

Instructions:

1. Preheat the oven to 375°F (190°C).

2. In a bowl, mix black beans, corn, diced bell pepper, and diced zucchini.

3. Warm the tortillas, then spoon the vegetable mixture onto each tortilla and roll it up.

4. Place the rolled tortillas in a baking dish, seam side down. Pour enchilada sauce over them and top with shredded cheese.

5. Bake for 20-25 minutes or until the cheese is melted and bubbly.

Nutrition Information:

- Calories: 280
- Protein: 12g
- Carbohydrates: 40g
- Fat: 8g
- Fiber: 8g
- Sugar: 5g
- Portion Size: 2 enchiladas

Garlic and Herb Roasted Vegetables with Tofu

Ingredients:

- 1 block extra-firm tofu (pressed and cubed)

- 3 cups mixed vegetables (broccoli, bell peppers, carrots)
- 2 tablespoons olive oil
- 3 cloves garlic (minced)
- 1 teaspoon dried thyme
- 1 teaspoon dried rosemary
- Salt and pepper to taste

Instructions:

1. Preheat the oven to 400°F (200°C).
2. In a bowl, toss cubed tofu and mixed vegetables with olive oil, minced garlic, dried thyme, dried rosemary, salt, and pepper.
3. Spread the mixture on a baking sheet and roast for 25-30 minutes, stirring halfway through.

Nutrition Information:

- Calories: 280
- Protein: 18g
- Carbohydrates: 20g
- Fat: 15g
- Fiber: 8g

- Sugar: 5g

- Portion Size: 1 cup

Stuffed Bell Peppers with Ground Turkey

Ingredients:

- 4 bell peppers (halved and seeds removed)

- 1 pound ground turkey

- 1 cup cooked quinoa

- 1 can (14 oz) diced tomatoes (drained)

- 1 cup black beans (rinsed and drained)

- 1 teaspoon cumin

- 1 teaspoon chili powder

- 1/2 cup shredded cheese (cheddar or Mexican blend)

Instructions:

1. Preheat the oven to 375°F (190°C).

2. In a skillet, cook ground turkey until browned. Add cooked quinoa, diced tomatoes, black beans, cumin, and chili powder. Mix well.

3. Stuff each bell pepper half with the turkey and quinoa mixture.

4. Sprinkle shredded cheese on top and bake for 25-30 minutes.

Nutrition Information:

- Calories: 320
- Protein: 24g
- Carbohydrates: 30g
- Fat: 12g
- Fiber: 7g
- Sugar: 5g
- Portion Size: 2 pepper halves

Shrimp and Vegetable Stir-Fry with Brown Rice

Ingredients:

- 1 pound shrimp (peeled and deveined)
- 2 cups mixed vegetables (broccoli, snap peas, carrots)
- 1 tablespoon soy sauce (low-sodium)

- 1 tablespoon oyster sauce
- 1 teaspoon sesame oil
- 2 cloves garlic (minced)
- 1 cup cooked brown rice

Instructions:

1. In a wok or skillet, heat sesame oil and sauté minced garlic.
2. Add shrimp and stir-fry until pink. Add mixed vegetables and continue to stir-fry.
3. Pour soy sauce and oyster sauce over the mixture, tossing to coat evenly.
4. Serve over a bed of cooked brown rice.

Nutrition Information:

- Calories: 280
- Protein: 22g
- Carbohydrates: 30g
- Fat: 8g
- Fiber: 5g
- Sugar: 3g
- Portion Size: 1 cup stir-fry with rice

Lemon Garlic Tilapia with Asparagus

Ingredients:

- 4 tilapia fillets

- 1 lemon (zested and juiced)

- 3 cloves garlic (minced)

- 2 tablespoons olive oil

- 1 bunch asparagus (trimmed)

- Salt and pepper to taste

Instructions:

1. Preheat the oven to 400°F (200°C).

2. In a small bowl, mix lemon zest, lemon juice, minced garlic, and olive oil.

3. Place tilapia fillets and trimmed asparagus on a baking sheet. Drizzle the lemon-garlic mixture over them.

4. Bake for 15-20 minutes or until tilapia is cooked through.

5. Season with salt and pepper before serving.

Nutrition Information:

- Calories: 220

- Protein: 30g

- Carbohydrates: 5g

- Fat: 9g

- Fiber: 2g

- Sugar: 2g

- Portion Size: 1 tilapia fillet with asparagus

Quinoa and Vegetable Casserole

Ingredients:

- 1 cup quinoa (cooked)

- 1 zucchini (diced)

- 1 bell pepper (chopped)

- 1 cup cherry tomatoes (halved)

- 1 cup spinach (chopped)

- 1/2 cup feta cheese (crumbled)

- 3 eggs

- 1 cup milk (or non-dairy alternative)

Instructions:

1. Preheat the oven to 375°F (190°C).

2. In a bowl, combine cooked quinoa, diced zucchini, chopped bell pepper, cherry tomatoes, chopped spinach, and crumbled feta cheese.

3. In a separate bowl, whisk eggs and milk. Pour over the quinoa and vegetable mixture.

4. Transfer the mixture to a baking dish and bake for 25-30 minutes or until set.

Nutrition Information:

- Calories: 280
- Protein: 15g
- Carbohydrates: 30g
- Fat: 12g
- Fiber: 5g
- Sugar: 6g
- Portion Size: 1 cup

Chicken and Broccoli Alfredo with Whole Wheat Pasta

Ingredients:

- 1 pound whole wheat pasta

- 1 pound chicken breast (sliced)
- 2 cups broccoli florets
- 2 tablespoons olive oil
- 2 cloves garlic (minced)
- 1 cup low-fat Alfredo sauce
- Salt and pepper to taste
- Grated Parmesan cheese for garnish

Instructions:

1. Cook whole wheat pasta according to package instructions. Drain and set aside.
2. In a skillet, heat olive oil and sauté minced garlic until fragrant.
3. Add sliced chicken and cook until browned. Add broccoli florets and continue cooking until chicken is cooked through.
4. Stir in low-fat Alfredo sauce and cooked pasta. Toss until well combined.
5. Season with salt and pepper. Garnish with grated Parmesan cheese before serving.

Nutrition Information:

- Calories: 400

- Protein: 30g

- Carbohydrates: 40g

- Fat: 15g

- Fiber: 6g

- Sugar: 3g

- Portion Size: 1.5 cups

Mediterranean Stuffed Chicken Breast

Ingredients:

- 4 chicken breasts

- 1 cup cherry tomatoes (halved)

- 1/2 cup Kalamata olives (pitted and sliced)

- 1/2 cup feta cheese (crumbled)

- 2 tablespoons olive oil

- 1 teaspoon dried oregano

- Salt and pepper to taste

Instructions:

1. Preheat the oven to 375°F (190°C).

2. In a bowl, mix cherry tomatoes, sliced Kalamata olives, crumbled feta cheese, olive oil, dried oregano, salt, and pepper.

3. Cut a pocket into each chicken breast and stuff with the Mediterranean mixture.

4. Place stuffed chicken breasts on a baking sheet and bake for 25-30 minutes.

Nutrition Information:

- Calories: 320
- Protein: 35g
- Carbohydrates: 5g
- Fat: 18g
- Fiber: 2g
- Sugar: 2g
- Portion Size: 1 stuffed chicken breast

Sweet and Sour Tofu with Cauliflower Rice

Ingredients:

- 1 block extra-firm tofu (cubed)
- 1 cup pineapple chunks
- 1 bell pepper (sliced)
- 1 cup snap peas
- 1/4 cup low-sodium soy sauce
- 2 tablespoons rice vinegar
- 2 tablespoons honey
- 1 tablespoon cornstarch
- 1 tablespoon vegetable oil
- Cauliflower rice (cooked)

Instructions:

1. In a bowl, whisk together soy sauce, rice vinegar, honey, and cornstarch to create the sauce.
2. In a skillet, heat vegetable oil and stir-fry cubed tofu until golden.
3. Add pineapple chunks, sliced bell pepper, and snap peas to the skillet. Stir-fry until vegetables are tender-crisp.

4. Pour the sweet and sour sauce over the tofu and vegetables. Stir until well-coated.

5. Serve over a bed of cooked cauliflower rice.

Nutrition Information:

- Calories: 280

- Protein: 15g

- Carbohydrates: 40g

- Fat: 8g

- Fiber: 5g

- Sugar: 20g

- Portion Size: 1 cup

Turkey and Sweet Potato Chili

Ingredients:

- 1 pound ground turkey

- 2 sweet potatoes (peeled and diced)

- 1 can (15 oz) black beans (rinsed and drained)

- 1 can (14 oz) diced tomatoes

- 1 onion (chopped)

- 2 cloves garlic (minced)

- 1 tablespoon chili powder

- 1 teaspoon cumin

- Salt and pepper to taste

Instructions:

1. In a large pot, cook ground turkey until browned. Add chopped onion and minced garlic.

2. Add diced sweet potatoes, black beans, diced tomatoes, chili powder, cumin, salt, and pepper to the pot. Stir well.

3. Simmer for 20-25 minutes or until sweet potatoes are tender.

4. Adjust seasoning if needed before serving.

Nutrition Information:

- Calories: 320

- Protein: 25g

- Carbohydrates: 35g

- Fat: 10g

- Fiber: 8g

- Sugar: 8g

- Portion Size: 1.5 cups

BBQ Grilled Veggie Skewers

Ingredients:

- 2 bell peppers (cut into chunks)
- 1 zucchini (sliced)
- 1 red onion (cut into wedges)
- 1 cup cherry tomatoes
- 1 cup button mushrooms
- 1 pound firm tofu (cubed)
- 1/2 cup barbecue sauce
- 2 tablespoons olive oil
- 1 teaspoon smoked paprika
- Salt and pepper to taste

Instructions:

1. Preheat the grill to medium-high heat.
2. In a bowl, mix barbecue sauce, olive oil, smoked paprika, salt, and pepper.
3. Thread bell pepper chunks, zucchini slices, red onion wedges, cherry tomatoes, mushrooms, and tofu cubes onto skewers.
4. Brush the veggie skewers with the barbecue sauce mixture.

5. Grill for 10-15 minutes, turning occasionally, until vegetables are charred and tofu is golden.

Nutrition Information:

- Calories: 250
- Protein: 15g
- Carbohydrates: 30g
- Fat: 10g
- Fiber: 8g
- Sugar: 15g
- Portion Size: 1 skewer

Chapter 5: Snacks and Appetizers

Welcome to Chapter 5, where we delve into a delightful array of snacks and appetizers designed with your taste buds and well-being in mind. These recipes are crafted to not only satisfy your cravings but also to provide a healthy option for those managing Type 1 diabetes. Packed with flavor and goodness, these snacks and appetizers are perfect for any occasion.

Hummus and Veggie Sticks

Ingredients:

- 1 cup chickpeas, drained and rinsed
- 2 tablespoons tahini
- 2 cloves garlic, minced
- 3 tablespoons olive oil
- 1 teaspoon cumin
- Salt and pepper to taste
- Assorted veggies for dipping (carrot sticks, cucumber, bell pepper)

Instructions:

1. In a food processor, blend chickpeas, tahini, garlic, olive oil, cumin, salt, and pepper until smooth.

2. Serve the hummus with an assortment of fresh vegetable sticks.

Nutrition Information:

- Calories: 120
- Protein: 4g
- Carbohydrates: 14g
- Fat: 6g
- Fiber: 4g
- Sugar: 2g
- Portion Size: 2 tablespoons hummus with veggies

Guacamole with Whole Wheat Pita Chips

Ingredients:

- 2 ripe avocados
- 1 tomato, diced
- 1/4 cup red onion, finely chopped

- 1 clove garlic, minced

- 1 lime, juiced

- Salt and pepper to taste

- Whole wheat pita, cut into triangles for dipping

Instructions:

1. Mash avocados in a bowl and add diced tomato, red onion, garlic, lime juice, salt, and pepper.
2. Mix well and serve with whole wheat pita chips.

Nutrition Information:

- Calories: 160

- Protein: 3g

- Carbohydrates: 18g

- Fat: 10g

- Fiber: 8g

- Sugar: 2g

- Portion Size: 1/2 cup guacamole with pita chips

Greek Yogurt and Berry Parfait

Ingredients:

- 1 cup Greek yogurt

- 1/2 cup mixed berries (strawberries, blueberries, raspberries)
- 2 tablespoons honey
- Granola for added crunch

Instructions:

1. In a glass or bowl, layer Greek yogurt, mixed berries, and a drizzle of honey.
2. Repeat the layers and top with granola.

Nutrition Information:

- Calories: 220
- Protein: 15g
- Carbohydrates: 30g
- Fat: 5g
- Fiber: 4g
- Sugar: 20g
- Portion Size: 1 cup parfait

Almond and Date Energy Balls

Ingredients:

- 1 cup almonds

- 1 cup dates, pitted

- 2 tablespoons chia seeds

- 1 tablespoon cocoa powder

- 1/2 teaspoon vanilla extract

- Pinch of salt

- Unsweetened shredded coconut for coating

Instructions:

1. In a food processor, blend almonds, dates, chia seeds, cocoa powder, vanilla extract, and salt until a sticky dough forms.

2. Roll the mixture into small balls and coat with shredded coconut.

Nutrition Information:

- Calories: 90

- Protein: 2g

- Carbohydrates: 10g

- Fat: 5g

- Fiber: 3g

- Sugar: 6g

- Portion Size: 2 energy balls

Edamame with Sea Salt

Ingredients:

- 2 cups edamame, steamed
- Sea salt to taste

Instructions:

1. Steam the edamame according to package instructions.
2. Sprinkle with sea salt and toss to coat.

Nutrition Information:

- Calories: 150
- Protein: 13g
- Carbohydrates: 9g
- Fat: 8g
- Fiber: 6g
- Sugar: 2g
- Portion Size: 1 cup edamame

Veggie and Cheese Skewers

Ingredients:

- Cherry tomatoes
- Cucumber, cut into chunks
- Bell peppers, assorted colors, cut into squares
- Mozzarella cheese, cubed
- Balsamic glaze for drizzling

Instructions:

1. Thread cherry tomatoes, cucumber chunks, bell pepper squares, and mozzarella cheese onto skewers.
2. Drizzle with balsamic glaze before serving.

Nutrition Information:

- Calories: 120
- Protein: 6g
- Carbohydrates: 8g
- Fat: 7g
- Fiber: 2g
- Sugar: 4g
- Portion Size: 2 skewers

Cottage Cheese and Pineapple Salsa

Ingredients:

- 1 cup low-fat cottage cheese
- 1 cup fresh pineapple, diced
- 1/4 cup red onion, finely chopped
- 1 jalapeño, seeded and minced
- Fresh cilantro, chopped
- Lime juice to taste

Instructions:

1. In a bowl, mix cottage cheese, diced pineapple, red onion, jalapeño, cilantro, and lime juice.
2. Refrigerate before serving.

Nutrition Information:

- Calories: 160
- Protein: 15g
- Carbohydrates: 20g
- Fat: 2g
- Fiber: 3g
- Sugar: 15g
- Portion Size: 1/2 cup serving

Apple Slices with Nut Butter

Ingredients:

- 2 apples, sliced
- Almond or peanut butter for dipping

Instructions:

1. Slice apples into wedges.
2. Dip apple slices into almond or peanut butter before enjoying.

Nutrition Information:

- Calories: 180
- Protein: 4g
- Carbohydrates: 26g
- Fat: 9g
- Fiber: 6g
- Sugar: 18g
- Portion Size: 1 medium apple with 2 tablespoons nut butter

Roasted Chickpeas with Cumin

Ingredients:

- 2 cups canned chickpeas, drained and rinsed
- 2 tablespoons olive oil
- 1 teaspoon ground cumin
- 1/2 teaspoon smoked paprika
- Salt to taste

Instructions:

1. Preheat the oven to 400°F (200°C).
2. Toss chickpeas with olive oil, cumin, paprika, and salt. Roast until crispy, about 25-30 minutes.

Nutrition Information:

- Calories: 200
- Protein: 8g
- Carbohydrates: 30g
- Fat: 7g
- Fiber: 8g
- Sugar: 5g
- Portion Size: 1/2 cup serving

Caprese Skewers with Balsamic Glaze

Ingredients:

- Cherry tomatoes
- Fresh mozzarella balls
- Fresh basil leaves
- Balsamic glaze for drizzling

Instructions:

1. Thread cherry tomatoes, mozzarella balls, and fresh basil leaves onto skewers.
2. Drizzle with balsamic glaze before serving.

Nutrition Information:

- Calories: 160
- Protein: 8g
- Carbohydrates: 5g
- Fat: 12g
- Fiber: 1g
- Sugar: 3g
- Portion Size: 2 skewers

Trail Mix with Nuts and Dried Fruit

Ingredients:

- 1 cup mixed nuts (almonds, walnuts, cashews)
- 1/2 cup dried fruit (apricots, cranberries, raisins)
- 1/4 cup dark chocolate chips

Instructions:

1. Combine mixed nuts, dried fruit, and dark chocolate chips in a bowl.
2. Mix well and portion into snack-sized servings.

Nutrition Information:

- Calories: 220
- Protein: 6g
- Carbohydrates: 20g
- Fat: 15g
- Fiber: 4g
- Sugar: 10g
- Portion Size: 1/4 cup serving

Whole Grain Crackers with Smoked Salmon

Ingredients:

- Whole grain crackers
- Smoked salmon slices
- Cream cheese
- Fresh dill for garnish

Instructions:

1. Spread cream cheese on whole grain crackers.
2. Top with smoked salmon slices and garnish with fresh dill.

Nutrition Information:

- Calories: 180
- Protein: 10g
- Carbohydrates: 15g
- Fat: 8g
- Fiber: 3g
- Sugar: 2g
- Portion Size: 6 crackers with salmon

Kale Chips with Parmesan

Ingredients:

- 1 bunch kale, stems removed and torn into pieces
- 2 tablespoons olive oil
- 1/4 cup grated Parmesan cheese
- Salt and pepper to taste

Instructions:

1. Preheat the oven to 350°F (175°C).
2. Toss kale with olive oil, Parmesan, salt, and pepper. Bake until crispy, about 15 minutes.

Nutrition Information:

- Calories: 120
- Protein: 5g
- Carbohydrates: 8g
- Fat: 8g
- Fiber: 2g
- Sugar: 1g
- Portion Size: 1 cup serving

Greek Salad Lettuce Wraps

Ingredients:

- Romaine lettuce leaves
- Greek salad mixture (cucumber, cherry tomatoes, feta cheese, olives)
- Greek dressing

Instructions:

1. Fill each lettuce leaf with the Greek salad mixture.
2. Drizzle with Greek dressing and serve as wraps.

Nutrition Information:

- Calories: 160
- Protein: 6g
- Carbohydrates: 12g
- Fat: 10g
- Fiber: 3g
- Sugar: 5g
- Portion Size: 2 lettuce wraps

Mini Turkey and Quinoa Meatballs

Ingredients:

- 1/2 pound ground turkey
- 1/2 cup cooked quinoa
- 1/4 cup grated Parmesan cheese
- 1 egg
- 1 teaspoon Italian seasoning
- Marinara sauce for dipping

Instructions:

1. Preheat the oven to 375°F (190°C).
2. In a bowl, mix ground turkey, cooked quinoa, Parmesan cheese, egg, and Italian seasoning. Form mini meatballs and bake until cooked through.
3. Serve with marinara sauce for dipping.

Nutrition Information:

- Calories: 180
- Protein: 15g
- Carbohydrates: 10g
- Fat: 8g
- Fiber: 2g

- Sugar: 1g
- Portion Size: 4 meatballs

Chapter 6: Desserts

Welcome to the delightful world of Chapter 6, where we explore scrumptious desserts tailored for those with a sweet tooth and a mindful approach to health. Indulge in these guilt-free creations that not only satisfy your cravings but also align with the principles of a diabetes-friendly lifestyle. Each recipe is crafted with care, focusing on wholesome ingredients and delightful flavors.

Berry and Yogurt Popsicles

Ingredients:

- 1 cup mixed berries (strawberries, blueberries, raspberries)
- 1 cup plain Greek yogurt
- 2 tablespoons honey

Instructions:

1. Blend the mixed berries until smooth.
2. In a bowl, mix the blended berries with Greek yogurt and honey.

3. Pour the mixture into popsicle molds.

4. Freeze for at least 4 hours.

5. Enjoy!

Nutrition Information:

- Calories: 80

- Protein: 5g

- Carbohydrates: 15g

- Fat: 1g

- Fiber: 2g

- Sugar: 11g

- Portion Size: 1 popsicle

Dark Chocolate-Dipped Strawberries

Ingredients:

- 1 cup dark chocolate chips
- 1 pint fresh strawberries, washed and dried

Instructions:

1. Melt dark chocolate in a heatproof bowl.

2. Dip each strawberry into the melted chocolate, coating it partially.

3. Place on a parchment-lined tray.

4. Allow the chocolate to set.

5. Indulge in these decadent treats!

Nutrition Information:

- Calories: 45

- Protein: 1g

- Carbohydrates: 8g

- Fat: 2g

- Fiber: 2g

- Sugar: 5g

- Portion Size: 3 strawberries

Banana and Walnut Muffins

Ingredients:

- 2 ripe bananas, mashed

- 1/4 cup melted coconut oil

- 1/2 cup honey

- 1 teaspoon vanilla extract

- 2 eggs

- 1 3/4 cups whole wheat flour

- 1/2 teaspoon baking soda

- 1/4 teaspoon salt
- 1/2 cup chopped walnuts

Instructions:

1. Preheat oven to 325°F (165°C).
2. Mix bananas, coconut oil, honey, vanilla, and eggs in a bowl.
3. In another bowl, whisk flour, baking soda, and salt.
4. Combine wet and dry ingredients, then fold in walnuts.
5. Pour into muffin cups and bake for 20-25 minutes.
6. Let cool before serving.

Nutrition Information:

- Calories: 180
- Protein: 4g
- Carbohydrates: 25g
- Fat: 8g
- Fiber: 3g
- Sugar: 12g
- Portion Size: 1 muffin

Greek Yogurt and Honey Frozen Cups

Ingredients:

- 2 cups plain Greek yogurt
- 1/4 cup honey
- 1 teaspoon vanilla extract

Instructions:

1. Mix Greek yogurt, honey, and vanilla in a bowl.
2. Spoon the mixture into cupcake liners in a muffin tin.
3. Freeze for at least 3 hours.
4. Remove from liners and enjoy!

Nutrition Information:

- Calories: 100
- Protein: 8g
- Carbohydrates: 14g
- Fat: 2g
- Fiber: 0g
- Sugar: 12g
- Portion Size: 1 frozen cup

Baked Apple with Cinnamon

Ingredients:

- 2 apples, cored and sliced
- 1 teaspoon cinnamon
- 1 tablespoon honey

Instructions:

1. Preheat oven to 375°F (190°C).
2. Toss apple slices with cinnamon and honey.
3. Bake for 20-25 minutes until tender.
4. Serve warm.

Nutrition Information:

- Calories: 90
- Protein: 0g
- Carbohydrates: 24g
- Fat: 0g
- Fiber: 4g
- Sugar: 19g
- Portion Size: 1 apple

Avocado Chocolate Mousse

Ingredients:

- 2 ripe avocados
- 1/2 cup unsweetened cocoa powder
- 1/4 cup maple syrup
- 1 teaspoon vanilla extract
- Pinch of salt

Instructions:

1. Blend avocados until smooth.
2. Add cocoa powder, maple syrup, vanilla, and salt. Blend until creamy.
3. Chill in the refrigerator for 2 hours.
4. Serve chilled.

Nutrition Information:

- Calories: 150
- Protein: 3g
- Carbohydrates: 20g
- Fat: 10g
- Fiber: 7g
- Sugar: 9g

- Portion Size: 1/2 cup

Almond Flour Blueberry Cookies

Ingredients:

- 1 cup almond flour
- 1/4 cup coconut oil, melted
- 1/4 cup maple syrup
- 1 teaspoon vanilla extract
- 1/2 cup fresh blueberries

Instructions:

1. Preheat oven to 350°F (175°C).
2. Mix almond flour, melted coconut oil, maple syrup, and vanilla.
3. Gently fold in blueberries.
4. Spoon onto a baking sheet and bake for 12-15 minutes.
5. Let cool before enjoying.

Nutrition Information:

- Calories: 90
- Protein: 2g

- Carbohydrates: 8g
- Fat: 6g
- Fiber: 1g
- Sugar: 5g
- Portion Size: 2 cookies

Mango and Coconut Chia Pudding

Ingredients:

- 1/4 cup chia seeds
- 1 cup coconut milk
- 1 teaspoon honey
- 1/2 cup diced mango

Instructions:

1. Mix chia seeds, coconut milk, and honey in a jar. Stir well.
2. Refrigerate overnight.
3. Layer with diced mango before serving.

Nutrition Information:

- Calories: 120
- Protein: 3g

- Carbohydrates: 14g
- Fat: 7g
- Fiber: 6g
- Sugar: 7g
- Portion Size: 1/2 cup

Pumpkin Pie Smoothie

Ingredients:

- 1/2 cup canned pumpkin puree
- 1/2 banana
- 1 cup almond milk
- 1/2 teaspoon pumpkin spice
- 1 tablespoon maple syrup

Instructions:

1. Blend pumpkin puree, banana, almond milk, pumpkin spice, and maple syrup until smooth.
2. Pour into a glass and enjoy!

Nutrition Information:

- Calories: 120
- Protein: 2g

- Carbohydrates: 20g
- Fat: 4g
- Fiber: 4g
- Sugar: 12g
- Portion Size: 1 smoothie

Mixed Berry Sorbet

Ingredients:

- 2 cups mixed berries (strawberries, blueberries, raspberries)
- 1/4 cup honey
- 1 tablespoon lemon juice

Instructions:

1. Blend berries, honey, and lemon juice until smooth.
2. Pour into a shallow dish and freeze for 4 hours.
3. Scoop and serve!

Nutrition Information:

- Calories: 70
- Protein: 1g
- Carbohydrates: 18g

- Fat: 0g
- Fiber: 4g
- Sugar: 14g
- Portion Size: 1/2 cup

Quinoa and Berry Parfait

Ingredients:

- 1 cup cooked quinoa, cooled
- 1 cup mixed berries (strawberries, blueberries, raspberries)
- 1 cup Greek yogurt
- 2 tablespoons honey

Instructions:

1. In a glass, layer quinoa, mixed berries, and Greek yogurt.
2. Drizzle with honey.
3. Repeat layers.
4. Top with a sprinkle of berries.
5. Serve chilled.

Nutrition Information:

- Calories: 220
- Protein: 12g
- Carbohydrates: 38g
- Fat: 3g
- Fiber: 6g
- Sugar: 18g
- Portion Size: 1 parfait

Cinnamon Baked Pears

Ingredients:

- 2 pears, halved and cored
- 1 teaspoon cinnamon
- 1 tablespoon honey

Instructions:

1. Preheat oven to 375°F (190°C).
2. Place pear halves on a baking sheet.
3. Sprinkle with cinnamon and drizzle with honey.
4. Bake for 20-25 minutes.
5. Serve warm.

Nutrition Information:

- Calories: 90
- Protein: 1g
- Carbohydrates: 24g
- Fat: 0g
- Fiber: 6g
- Sugar: 15g
- Portion Size: 1 pear

Coconut Flour Chocolate Cake

Ingredients:

- 1/2 cup coconut flour
- 1/4 cup cocoa powder
- 1/2 teaspoon baking soda
- 1/4 teaspoon salt
- 4 eggs
- 1/2 cup coconut oil, melted
- 1/2 cup honey
- 1 teaspoon vanilla extract

Instructions:

1. Preheat oven to 350°F (175°C).

2. In a bowl, mix coconut flour, cocoa powder, baking soda, and salt.

3. In another bowl, whisk eggs, coconut oil, honey, and vanilla.

4. Combine wet and dry ingredients.

5. Pour into a greased cake pan and bake for 25-30 minutes.

6. Allow to cool before slicing.

Nutrition Information:

- Calories: 180
- Protein: 4g
- Carbohydrates: 20g
- Fat: 10g
- Fiber: 3g
- Sugar: 13g
- Portion Size: 1 slice

Peanut Butter and Banana Ice Cream

Ingredients:

- 2 ripe bananas, sliced and frozen
- 2 tablespoons peanut butter
- 1/4 cup almond milk

Instructions:

1. Blend frozen banana slices, peanut butter, and almond milk until creamy.
2. Freeze for 2 hours.
3. Scoop and enjoy!

Nutrition Information:

- Calories: 150
- Protein: 3g
- Carbohydrates: 26g
- Fat: 5g
- Fiber: 4g
- Sugar: 14g
- Portion Size: 1/2 cup

Lemon Poppy Seed Energy Bites

Ingredients:

- 1 cup rolled oats
- 1/2 cup almond butter
- 1/4 cup honey
- Zest of 1 lemon
- 1 tablespoon poppy seeds

Instructions:

1. In a bowl, mix rolled oats, almond butter, honey, lemon zest, and poppy seeds.
2. Form into bite-sized balls.
3. Refrigerate for at least 30 minutes.
4. Enjoy these energy-packed bites!

Nutrition Information:

- Calories: 90
- Protein: 3g
- Carbohydrates: 12g
- Fat: 4g
- Sugar: 5g
- Portion Size: 2 bites

Chapter 7: Smoothies

In Chapter 7, we present an ensemble of Smoothies that effortlessly blend health and taste. From the vibrant hues of the Green Power Smoothie to the comforting richness of the Coffee and Almond Protein Smoothie, each recipe is a unique ode to wellness. Let's dive into the delightful universe of these smooth concoctions that make every sip a moment of nourishment.

Green Power Smoothie

Ingredients:

- 1 cup fresh spinach leaves
- 1/2 cucumber, peeled and sliced
- 1 green apple, cored and chopped
- 1/2 lemon, juiced
- 1 cup water or coconut water
- Ice cubes (optional)

Instructions:

1. Combine spinach, cucumber, green apple, and lemon juice in a blender.
2. Add water or coconut water for desired consistency.
3. Blend until smooth.
4. Add ice cubes if desired and blend again.
5. Pour into a glass and enjoy!

Nutrition Information (per serving):

*   Calories: 90
*   Protein: 3g
*   Carbohydrates: 22g
*   Fat: 0.5g
*   Fiber: 5g
*   Sugar: 14g
*   Portion Size: 1 serving

Berry Blast Smoothie

Ingredients:

*   1 cup mixed berries (strawberries, blueberries, raspberries)
*   1 banana, peeled

- 1/2 cup Greek yogurt

- 1 tablespoon honey

- 1 cup almond milk

- Ice cubes (optional)

Instructions:

1. Combine mixed berries, banana, Greek yogurt, honey, and almond milk in a blender.

2. Blend until smooth.

3. Add ice cubes if desired and blend again.

4. Pour into a glass and savor the berry bliss!

Nutrition Information (per serving):

- Calories: 150

- Protein: 6g

- Carbohydrates: 30g

- Fat: 2g

- Fiber: 5g

- Sugar: 20g

- Portion Size: 1 serving

Mango Tango Smoothie

Ingredients:

- 1 cup chopped mango
- 1/2 cup pineapple chunks
- 1/2 cup orange juice
- 1/2 cup coconut milk
- 1 tablespoon chia seeds
- Ice cubes (optional)

Instructions:

1. Combine chopped mango, pineapple chunks, orange juice, coconut milk, and chia seeds in a blender.
2. Blend until smooth.
3. Add ice cubes if desired and blend again.
4. Pour into a glass and relish the tropical delight!

Nutrition Information (per serving):

- Calories: 180
- Protein: 3g
- Carbohydrates: 35g
- Fat: 5g
- Fiber: 6g

- Sugar: 25g
- Portion Size: 1 serving

Spinach and Pineapple Smoothie

Ingredients:

- 1 cup fresh spinach leaves
- 1 cup pineapple chunks
- 1 banana, peeled
- 1/2 cup coconut water
- 1 tablespoon flaxseeds
- Ice cubes (optional)

Instructions:

1. Combine fresh spinach, pineapple chunks, banana, coconut water, and flaxseeds in a blender.
2. Blend until smooth.
3. Add ice cubes if desired and blend again.
4. Pour into a glass and revel in the tropical goodness!

Nutrition Information (per serving):

- Calories: 120
- Protein: 3.5g

- Carbohydrates: 28g
- Fat: 2g
- Fiber: 6g
- Sugar: 15g
- Portion Size: 1 serving

Chocolate Banana Protein Smoothie

Ingredients:

- 1 banana, peeled
- 2 tablespoons cocoa powder
- 1/2 cup Greek yogurt
- 1 scoop chocolate protein powder
- 1 cup almond milk
- Ice cubes (optional)

Instructions:

1. Combine banana, cocoa powder, Greek yogurt, chocolate protein powder, and almond milk in a blender.
2. Blend until smooth.
3. Add ice cubes if desired and blend again.

4. Pour into a glass and enjoy the chocolaty protein goodness!

Nutrition Information (per serving):

- Calories: 220
- Protein: 20g
- Carbohydrates: 30g
- Fat: 4g
- Fiber: 7g
- Sugar: 15g
- Portion Size: 1 serving

Avocado and Kale Smoothie

Ingredients:

- 1/2 avocado, peeled and pitted
- 1 cup kale leaves, stems removed
- 1/2 banana, peeled
- 1 tablespoon honey
- 1 cup coconut water
- Ice cubes (optional)

Instructions:

1. Combine avocado, kale leaves, banana, honey, and coconut water in a blender.
2. Blend until smooth.
3. Add ice cubes if desired and blend again.
4. Pour into a glass and relish the creamy green goodness!

Nutrition Information (per serving):

- Calories: 160
- Protein: 3g
- Carbohydrates: 25g
- Fat: 8g
- Fiber: 7g
- Sugar: 15g
- Portion Size: 1 serving

Tropical Paradise Smoothie

Ingredients:

- 1 cup mango chunks
- 1/2 cup pineapple chunks
- 1/2 cup coconut milk

- 1/2 cup orange juice
- 1 tablespoon shredded coconut
- Ice cubes (optional)

Instructions:

1. Combine mango chunks, pineapple chunks, coconut milk, orange juice, and shredded coconut in a blender.
2. Blend until smooth.
3. Add ice cubes if desired and blend again.
4. Pour into a glass and transport yourself to a tropical paradise!

Nutrition Information (per serving):

- Calories: 190
- Protein: 2.5g
- Carbohydrates: 35g
- Fat: 6g
- Fiber: 4g
- Sugar: 25g
- Portion Size: 1 serving

Blueberry Almond Butter Smoothie

Ingredients:

- 1 cup blueberries
- 1 banana, peeled
- 2 tablespoons almond butter
- 1/2 cup Greek yogurt
- 1 cup almond milk
- Ice cubes (optional)

Instructions:

1. Combine blueberries, banana, almond butter, Greek yogurt, and almond milk in a blender.
2. Blend until smooth.
3. Add ice cubes if desired and blend again.
4. Pour into a glass and savor the nutty berry goodness!

Nutrition Information (per serving):

- Calories: 220
- Protein: 8g
- Carbohydrates: 30g
- Fat: 9g
- Fiber: 6g

- Sugar: 16g
- Portion Size: 1 serving

Cucumber Mint Refresh Smoothie

Ingredients:

- 1 cucumber, peeled and sliced
- 1/2 cup fresh mint leaves
- 1/2 lime, juiced
- 1/2 cup Greek yogurt
- 1 tablespoon honey
- Ice cubes (optional)

Instructions:

1. Combine cucumber, mint leaves, lime juice, Greek yogurt, and honey in a blender.
2. Blend until smooth.
3. Add ice cubes if desired and blend again.
4. Pour into a glass and experience the refreshing zing!

Nutrition Information (per serving):

- Calories: 100
- Protein: 4g

- Carbohydrates: 20g
- Fat: 1g
- Fiber: 3g
- Sugar: 15g
- Portion Size: 1 serving

Orange Creamsicle Smoothie

Ingredients:

- 1 cup orange segments
- 1/2 cup Greek yogurt
- 1/2 cup almond milk
- 1 tablespoon honey
- 1 teaspoon vanilla extract
- Ice cubes (optional)

Instructions:

1. Combine orange segments, Greek yogurt, almond milk, honey, and vanilla extract in a blender.
2. Blend until smooth.
3. Add ice cubes if desired and blend again.
4. Pour into a glass and relish the nostalgic flavor of an orange creamsicle!

Nutrition Information (per serving):

- Calories: 130
- Protein: 5g
- Carbohydrates: 25g
- Fat: 2.5g
- Fiber: 4g
- Sugar: 18g
- Portion Size: 1 serving

Kiwi and Strawberry Delight Smoothie

Ingredients:

- 2 kiwis, peeled and sliced
- 1 cup strawberries, hulled
- 1/2 cup coconut water
- 1/2 cup Greek yogurt
- 1 tablespoon chia seeds
- Ice cubes (optional)

Instructions:

1. Combine kiwis, strawberries, coconut water, Greek yogurt, and chia seeds in a blender.
2. Blend until smooth.
3. Add ice cubes if desired and blend again.
4. Pour into a glass and enjoy the delightful fusion of kiwi and strawberry!

Nutrition Information (per serving):

- Calories: 150
- Protein: 4g
- Carbohydrates: 30g
- Fat: 3g
- Fiber: 7g
- Sugar: 18g
- Portion Size: 1 serving

Peanut Butter Banana Oat Smoothie

Ingredients:

- 1 banana, peeled
- 2 tablespoons peanut butter
- 1/4 cup rolled oats

- 1/2 cup Greek yogurt

- 1 cup almond milk

- Ice cubes (optional)

Instructions:

1. Combine banana, peanut butter, rolled oats, Greek yogurt, and almond milk in a blender.

2. Blend until smooth.

3. Add ice cubes if desired and blend again.

4. Pour into a glass and relish the creamy goodness of peanut butter and banana!

Nutrition Information (per serving):

- Calories: 250

- Protein: 11g

- Carbohydrates: 30g

- Fat: 11g

- Fiber: 5g

- Sugar: 15g

- Portion Size: 1 serving

Raspberry Coconut Chia Smoothie

Ingredients:

- 1 cup raspberries
- 1/2 cup coconut milk
- 1/2 cup Greek yogurt
- 1 tablespoon chia seeds
- 1 tablespoon honey
- Ice cubes (optional)

Instructions:

1. Combine raspberries, coconut milk, Greek yogurt, chia seeds, and honey in a blender.
2. Blend until smooth.
3. Add ice cubes if desired and blend again.
4. Pour into a glass and relish the delightful combination of raspberry and coconut with the added crunch of chia seeds!

Nutrition Information (per serving):

- Calories: 180
- Protein: 5g
- Carbohydrates: 25g

- Fat: 8g

- Fiber: 9g

- Sugar: 15g

- Portion Size: 1 serving

Watermelon Mint Cooler Smoothie

Ingredients:

- 2 cups watermelon cubes

- 1/4 cup fresh mint leaves

- 1/2 lime, juiced

- 1/2 cup coconut water

- 1 tablespoon agave syrup

- Ice cubes (optional)

Instructions:

1. Combine watermelon cubes, fresh mint leaves, lime juice, coconut water, and agave syrup in a blender.

2. Blend until smooth.

3. Add ice cubes if desired and blend again.

4. Pour into a glass and experience the refreshing coolness of watermelon and mint!

Nutrition Information (per serving):

- Calories: 100
- Protein: 2g
- Carbohydrates: 25g
- Fat: 0.5g
- Fiber: 2g
- Sugar: 20g
- Portion Size: 1 serving

Coffee and Almond Protein Smoothie

Ingredients:

- 1/2 cup brewed coffee, cooled
- 1/2 banana, peeled
- 1 scoop vanilla protein powder
- 1 tablespoon almond butter
- 1/2 cup almond milk
- Ice cubes (optional)

Instructions:

1. Combine brewed coffee, banana, vanilla protein powder, almond butter, and almond milk in a blender.
2. Blend until smooth.
3. Add ice cubes if desired and blend again.
4. Pour into a glass and relish the energizing combination of coffee and almond protein!

Nutrition Information (per serving):

- Calories: 200
- Protein: 15g
- Carbohydrates: 20g
- Fat: 9g
- Fiber: 4g
- Sugar: 8g
- Portion Size: 1 serving

CONCLUSION

In concluding this "Type 1 Diabetes Cookbook for Beginners," we embark on more than just a culinary adventure; we embark on a journey towards a healthier, more vibrant life. Throughout the pages of this book, we've not only explored flavorful recipes but also delved into the intricacies of managing Type 1 Diabetes with a focus on nourishment.

As we bid farewell, remember that this is not just the end of a cookbook but the beginning of a newfound relationship with food—one that nourishes both body and soul. The 30-day meal plan serves as a launchpad, offering structure and variety to your daily diet, establishing healthy habits that can be sustained for a lifetime.

In each chapter, from the wholesome breakfasts that greet your mornings to the satisfying dinners that close your day, we've curated a symphony of flavors that dance in harmony with diabetes management. The snacks, desserts, and smoothies are not mere indulgences but crafted delights, ensuring that your journey is not just about sustenance but also about relishing every bite.

This book is not just a collection of recipes; it's a testament to the power of informed choices, thoughtful preparation, and the joy that comes from a well-balanced plate. Embrace the simplicity of a well-roasted vegetable and the richness of a carefully curated smoothie, for in these moments lies the essence of a mindful and healthful lifestyle.

As you navigate your way through these recipes, remember that flexibility is key. Feel free to swap ingredients, adjust portions, and make each dish your own. Cooking, after all, is an art, and you are the artist shaping your own culinary masterpiece.

In closing, let this cookbook be your companion, guiding you through the delicious realms of balanced nutrition. Let it be a reminder that managing Type 1 Diabetes isn't about restriction but about empowerment—empowerment to create, savor, and celebrate the vibrant tapestry of flavors that life has to offer.

Here's to a future filled with nourishing meals, thriving health, and the joy that comes from knowing you have the tools to make every bite count. May your culinary journey be both satisfying and inspiring, echoing the sentiments of a life well-lived—one delicious recipe at a time.